40 Super Food & Super Smoothie Recipes For Better Health

Feel Amazing, Lose Weight, and Gain Unlimited Energy

Ariana Hunter

© 2015

Copyright © All rights reserved. This book or any portion thereof may not be reproduced or used in any manner whatsoever without the express written permission of the publisher, except for brief quotations.

Disclaimer:

This book is not intended as a substitute for the medical advice of physicians. The reader should regularly consult a physician in matters relating to his/her health and particularly with respect to any symptoms that may require diagnosis or medical attention.

Table of Contents

- **INTRODUCTION** 3
- **GREEN SMOOTHIES** 4
  - Kale and Banana Smoothie 5
    - Super Clean and Super Green Smoothie 6
  - The Hempy 7
    - Berry Chlorella 8
- **DETOX SMOOTHIES** 9
  - Cacao Acai Detox 10
- The Fruity Lemongrass Smoothie 11
  - Kombucha Smoothie 12
- Kiwi Detox Smoothie 13
- **FAT BURNERS** 14
  - Orange and Oats Shake 15
- Hibiscus and Mulberry Fat Burner 16
  - Tropical Coconut Fat Burning Smoothie 17
- Dated Smoothie 18
- Coconut Coffee Smoothie 19
- **FOR THE TASTE** 20
  - Sweetest Breakfast 21
- Smooth and Fruity Italian Ice 22
  - Strawberry-Banana Soy Smoothie 23
- Peanut Butter Blast 24
  - Creamy Piña Colada 25
- Multi-Melon Protein Smoothie 26
- **SUPERFOODS** 27
- **BREAKFAST** 28
  - Banana Pancakes and Berries 29
- Garbanzo Pancakes 30
  - Sweet and Creamy Vanilla Multi-grain Hot Cereal 31
- Crispy Eggplant Bacon 32
- **SNACK** 33
  - Paleo Avocado in a Basket 34
- Seed Crunch Bunch 35
  - Sweet Nutty Snack Mix 36
- Quick Fruit Mix 37

LUNCH **38**
   Skillet Asparagus Salad with Goat Cheese 39
Refreshing Watermelon Salad 40
   Quinoa Chard Pilaf 41
Cabbage and Apple Salad 42
High Protein Egg and Salmon Sandwich 43
DINNER **44**
   Grilled Salmon with Spaghetti Squash and Pecan Salad 45
Tasty Tomato and Beet Salad 46
   Sweet Black Bean Burrito 47
Vegetarian Stuffed Red Bell Peppers 48
   Grilled Fiesta Fish Tacos with Lime-Yogurt Sauce 49
Mesquite Collard Greens 50
   Salmon Cakes with Chervil and Green Bean Salad 51

INTRODUCTION

Greetings! Let me start off by complimenting you for reading this eBook, and taking the initiative to better your health. If health is not your motivation for reading this book, then congratulations anyway. You are about to discover some of the best recipes and smoothies that are packed with many of the nutrients our body requires daily. You will come to find that these nutrients can be very useful to you, and hopefully you will want to get in the habit of incorporating these foods and recipes into your daily diet.

Today, there are a plethora of fad diets, exercise programs, magic beans, fairy dusts, mummification methods, etc. that sell you the delusion of and easy and healthy weight loss. But have you ever noticed that few of these products or programs stray away from the importance of how

It is safe to say that nothing works better than consuming the foods that come from the earth. Consuming highly organic, natural foods is always the BEST medicine for a healthy body. We as human beings are quite fortunate creatures. We have been graced with the presence of more likely "heaven sent" food to give us the body, temperament, and mind that we all secretly or openly desire.

Consider this book a small magnifying glass to some of the foods we hear about, see, or maybe even eat every day. This book comprised of recipes that highlight foods we often underestimate, and probably never heard of. My purpose is to help you gain a desire and a sense of excitement for eating foods that are natural, unrefined, and unprocessed.

So, start those blender engines and get your pots and pans ready!

Kale and Banana Smoothie

Kale is packed with many healthy vitamins. The mighty kale contains more iron than your everyday fleshy beef! This SUPER green has the ability lower cholesterol and strengthen your immune system. If you consume kale on a frequent basis, watch your digestive system change for the better.

Yield: One serving
Active Time: 5 minutes
Cooking Time: 0 minutes
Total Time: 5 minutes

Ingredients
2 cups kale, chopped
1 banana
1 tsp organic maple syrup
1 tbsp flax seed
½ cup light unsweetened soy milk

Directions
1. Blend together banana, kale, soy milk, flax seeds, and syrup in a blender until smooth.
2. Serve with ice.

Nutritional Information (Serving Size: 1 cup): Calories: 311, Calories from Fat: 66g, Saturated fat: 0.8g, Cholesterol: 0mg, Sodium: 110mg, Carbohydrates: 56.6g, Fiber: 10.1g, Protein: 12.2g

Super Clean and Super Green Smoothie

This tasty smoothie is packed with all of the superfoods you need on a daily basis. It's the perfect detox, and the perfect breakfast. Make breakfast mean something, and try this wonderful nutrient-packed smoothie.

Yield: One servings
Active Time: 5 minutes
Cooking Time: 0 minutes
Total Time: 5 minutes

Ingredients
1 cup kale, chopped
1 cup romaine, chopped
½ large green apple, chopped
½ cup large celery, chopped
1 large frozen banana, chopped (peel before freezing)
1 cup coconut water
2 tbsp lemon juice
½ tbsp chia seeds
2 tbsp fresh mint, chopped
2 tbsp Agave nectar
1 tbsp fresh parsley
1 tsp turmeric
1 tsp cayenne pepper
1 tsp cinnamon

Cooking Directions
1. Add all of the ingredients to the blender, and puree until all of the ingredients become completely smooth.
2. Pour into your favorite glass and enjoy!

Nutritional Information: Calories: 505, Total Fat: 4.4g, Saturated Fat: 0.7g, Cholesterol: 0mg, Sodium: 123mg, Carbohydrate: 120g, Dietary Fiber: 19g, Sugars: 80g, Protein: 9g

The Hempy

Your digestive system will thank you for this smoothie! The sweetness of the mango, strawberries, and tangerine together makes it hard to believe that this is a Super Green Smoothie. Hemp is a highly recommended vegetable protein that contains HIGH QUALITY dietary plant protein. Dietary protein is essential your body's healthy growth and maintenance.

Yield: One servings
Active Time: 5 minutes
Cooking Time: 0 minutes
Total Time: 5 minutes

Ingredients
2 tbsp hemp protein powder
¾ cup spinach, chopped
¾ cup fresh mango, cubed
½ cup strawberries, sliced
1 large celery stalk, chopped
½ cup tangerine
¼ cup parsley, chopped
Ice (optional)

Cooking Directions
1. Add all of the ingredients to the blender, and puree until all of the ingredients become completely smooth.
2. Pour into your favorite glass and enjoy!

(**If smoothie becomes too thick, feel free to add water in order to loosen the consistency.)

Nutritional Information: Calories: 219, Total Fat: 2g, Saturated Fat: 0g, Cholesterol: 0mg, Sodium: 86mg, Carbohydrate: 46g, Dietary Fiber: 13.5g, Protein: 7.1g

Berry Chlorella

If you haven't heard of chlorella, then you must've been hiding under a rock. Chlorella contains a noteworthy amount of protein, because it is mostly made up of the building-blocks of protein: AMINO ACIDS! Chlorella is also rich in iron and Vitamin B, D, A, and K. Amazing. Right? But what's really amazing is that you can get all of this by consuming only 1 teaspoon of this mean green vitamin-rich machine. Stop being an "algae" and try this smoothie. You'll love it benefits.

Yield: One servings
Active Time: 5 minutes
Cooking Time: 0 minutes
Total Time: 5 minutes

Ingredients
¾ cup pomegranate juice
½ cup papaya, chopped
1 large frozen banana, chopped (peel before freezing)
1 cup almond milk
2 tsp chlorella
Ice (optional)

Cooking Directions
1. Add all of the ingredients to the blender, and puree until all of the ingredients become completely smooth.
2. Pour into your favorite glass and enjoy!

Nutritional Information: Calories: 341, Total Fat: 3g, Saturated Fat: 0g, Cholesterol: 0mg, Sodium: 154mg, Carbohydrate: 46g, Dietary Fiber: 6g, Protein: 6g

Cacao Acai Detox

Cacao beans are rich in natural antioxidants called flavonoids. Flavonoids have the ability to destroy free radicals in your tissues and cells, and can also lower your risk of a number of diseases. This recipe is the perfect display of the power of cacao, and its power is heightened with the addition of other tasty superfoods.

Yield: Two Servings
Active Time: 5 minutes
Cooking Time: 0 minutes
Total Time: 5 minutes

Ingredients
½ cup fresh strawberries, sliced
⅛ cup Matcha green tea, powder
½ tbsp cacao fermented nibs
2 tbsp cacao powder
2 tbsp organic raw sun-dried goji berries
1 cup alfalfa sprouts
1 tsp acai powder
1 tbsp coconut peanut butter
1 cup coconut water
¼ avocado, chopped
1 tbsp organic raw honey
⅓ cup plain Greek yogurt
Ice (optional)

Cooking Directions
1. Add all of the ingredients to the blender, and puree until all of the ingredients become completely smooth.
2. Pour into your favorite glass and enjoy!

Nutritional Information: Calories: 386, Total Fat: 11g, Saturated Fat: 5g, Cholesterol: 0mg, Sodium: 56mg, Carbohydrate: 40g, Dietary Fiber: 10g, Protein: 11g

The Fruity Lemongrass Smoothie

Don't be fooled by the name. This herb is no kin of the citrusy and sour fruit that we all love so much. However, it does have a strong resemblance in smell and taste. Lemongrass has a powerful ability to assist in regulating a healthy digestion and helps kill those nasty little bacteria in the intestine and colon.

Yield: One Servings
Active Time: 5 minutes
Cooking Time: 0 minutes
Total Time: 5 minutes

Ingredients
1 large frozen banana, chopped (peel before freezing)
½ cup plain Greek yogurt
½ cup coconut milk
¼ cup organic rolled oats, cooked
1 tbsp ground flaxseeds
1 tbsp organic raw honey
½ cup Ice

Cooking Directions
1. Add all of the ingredients to the blender, and puree until all of the ingredients become completely smooth.
2. Pour into your favorite glass and enjoy!

Nutritional Information: Calories: 771, Total Fat: 22g, Saturated Fat: 9g, Cholesterol: 0mg, Sodium: 102mg, Carbohydrate: 80g, Dietary Fiber: 20g, Protein: 22g

Kombucha Smoothie

Did you know that our bodies are always in detox mode? Why not help your body get through that process easily by adding Kombucha to your diet. Kombucha is opulent in many of the enzymes and bacterial acids that are essential to the body's detoxification process. Ironically, our body naturally produces enzymes and bacterial acids, increasing your body's supply by consuming Kombucha tea, lightens the load on your pancreas and liver.

Yield: Two Servings
Active Time: 10 minutes
Cooking Time: 2 minutes
Total Time: 12 minutes

Ingredients
1 cup Gingerberry Kombucha
1 avocado, cored, peeled, and cubed
¾ cup fresh mango, cubed
½ cup blackberries
½ cup raspberries
2 tablespoons ground flax seeds
2 tbsp hemp protein powder
1 cup Ice

Cooking Directions
1. Pour Kombucha into the blender first. Dump all of the ingredients to the blender, and puree until all of the ingredients become completely smooth.
2. Pour into your favorite glass and enjoy!

Nutritional Information: Calories: 277, Total Fat: 17g, Saturated Fat: 2g, Cholesterol: 0mg, Sodium: 12mg, Carbohydrate: 24g, Dietary Fiber: 14g, Protein: 8g

Kiwi Detox Smoothie

This is a nutrient dense smoothie that will give you the energy you need to make it through the morning rush. It just so happens to be graced with the presence of kiwi, which is rich in disease fighting anti-oxidants. Kiwis have a special super power that allows them to bind and move those nasty toxins in your digestive tract out of the way. If consumed on a frequent basis will make constipation a thing of the past.

Yield: Two Servings
Active Time: 5 minutes
Cooking Time: 0 minutes
Total Time: 5 minutes

Ingredients
4 kiwi, peeled and quartered
2 tbsp hemp protein
½ cup hemp yogurt
1 cup Good Karma Flax Milk
½ Cup Blueberries
2 Ice Cubes

Directions
1. Add all of the ingredients to the blender, and puree until all of the ingredients become completely smooth.
2. Pour into your favorite glass and enjoy!

Nutritional Information: Calories: 240, Total Fat: 7g, Cholesterol: 222mg, Carbohydrates: 34g, Protein: 17g, Dietary Fiber: 7g

Orange and Oats Shake

The oats gives this shake the creaminess and thickness that is needed to top off your day. It's super filling and can be enjoyed for breakfast, lunch, dinner or dessert. Oats is the highlight of this smoothie, and their high fiber content is one of the nutrients that make oats an ideal ingredient in a fat burning smoothie. Oats are another food that is also rich in antioxidants.

Yield: Five servings
Active Time: 10 minutes
Cooking Time: 30 minutes
Total Time: 70 minutes

Ingredients
¼ cup orange juice, freshly squeezed
2 small tangerines
1 medium banana
¼ cup organic rolled oats, cooked
1 tbsp Agave nectar
1 cup fresh pineapple juice
2 quarts water
1 tsp ground cinnamon
1 cup Ice

Directions
1. Bring 2 quarts of water to a boil in a large pot. Reduce to medium-high heat and add oats. Allow oats to cook for 30 minutes, stirring sporadically. Remove from heat and allow oats to cool. Drain remaining liquid.
2. Add pineapple juice, oatmeal, orange juice, banana, ice, and sweetener to a blender. Blend mixture until it becomes smooth. Pour each serving into an 8 ounce serving glass, garnish glass with a pineapple wedge, and sprinkle cinnamon on top. Serve immediately and enjoy!

Nutritional Information (Serving Size: 1 cup): Calories: 170, Calories from Fat: 15, Saturated fat: 0g, Cholesterol: 0mg, Sodium: 15mg, Carbohydrates: 37g, Fiber: 3g, Protein: 4g

Hibiscus and Mulberry Fat Burner

Hibiscus tea is made from the calyces of the hibiscus flower, which are rich in antioxidants. The best part about this tea is that it helps decrease your appetite which can assist in weight loss. Mulberries has the ability to decrease the secretion of insulin, which will assist your body in burning stored fat at a higher rate and decrease fat storage from consuming a high amount of calories.

Yield: One Servings
Active Time: 10 minutes
Cooking Time: 2 minutes
Total Time: 12 minutes

Ingredients
1 large frozen banana, chopped (peel before freezing)
3 cups baby spinach, chopped
1 cup Hibiscus tea
1 cup mulberries
1 cup frozen blueberries
½ tsp ground cinnamon
1 cup Ice

Cooking Directions
1. Pour Hibiscus tea into the blender first. Dump all of the ingredients to the blender, and puree until all of the ingredients become completely smooth.
2. Pour into your favorite glass and enjoy!

Nutritional Information: Calories: 322, Total Fat: 2g, Saturated Fat: 0.3g, Cholesterol: 0mg, Sodium: 96mg, Carbohydrate: 78g, Dietary Fiber: 13g, Protein: 7g

Tropical Coconut Fat Burning Smoothie

The tasty COCONUT! It's one of the most delicious and versatile foods on the planet. Coconut has the ability to help speed up the metabolism, and source the body with instant energy. When you have more energy, you are inspired to move more. When you move more, you lose more (WEIGHT).

Yield: One Servings
Active Time: 10 minutes
Cooking Time: 2 minutes
Total Time: 12 minutes

Ingredients
1 large frozen banana, chopped (peel before freezing)
½ cup coconut water
½ cup coconut milk
2 large organic free range eggs
1 tablespoon unrefined extra-virgin coconut oil
½ cup fresh pineapple, cubed
Ice (optional)

Cooking Directions
1. Pour Hibiscus tea into the blender first. Dump all of the ingredients to the blender, and puree until all of the ingredients become completely smooth.
2. Pour into your favorite glass and enjoy!

Nutritional Information: Calories: 350, Total Fat: 17g, Saturated Fat: 16g, Cholesterol: 0mg, Sodium: 30mg, Carbohydrate: 49g, Dietary Fiber: 5g, Protein: 2g

Dated Smoothie

Dates are one those naturally sweet fruits that just make you want to come back for more. That is a good thing being that they contains some very useful nutrients. Dates have been known to supplement the intestine by providing it with nicotine. Now, I know throughout our lives, we've been told that consuming nicotine is bad. That's highly true when it comes to cigarettes. However, the nicotine in dates help cure and rid the intestines of any kind of sickness and disorder (constipation). A clean and clear intestine means that your body can help your burn off fat more efficiently.

Yield: Two servings
Active Time: 5 minutes
Cooking Time: 0 minutes
Total Time: 5 minutes

Ingredients
6 dates, pitted and chopped
2 tbsp natural peanut butter
2 cups low-fat milk
¾ cup plain non-fat yogurt
2 tbsp flax seed oil
1 tbsp rose flower water
¼ tsp ground cardamom

Directions
1. Add milk, yogurt, peanut butter, dates, water, flax seed oil, and cardamom to blender and blend until mixture is smooth and thick. Pour each serving into a single glass.

Nutritional Information (Serving Size: ½ of recipe): Calories: 340, Calories from Fat: 140g, Saturated fat: 2.5g, Cholesterol: 10mg, Sodium: 180mg, Carbohydrates: 42g, Fiber: 3g, Protein: 12g

Coconut Coffee Smoothie

Due to the plague of unhealthy coffee chains, coffee does not have as great of a reputation as it should.
Coffee can help people feel less tired and increase energy levels. The real kicker is that you find caffeine in almost every popular and highly advertised fat burning supplement. Why? Caffeine has been a proven fat burner, and also has the ability to increase your metabolic rate. So, enjoy this smoothie with a nice cup of coffee to increase the fat burning affects.

Yield: Two Servings
Active Time: 5 minutes
Cooking Time: 0 minutes
Total Time: 5 minutes

Ingredients
1 cup brewed coffee, cold
2 tbsp organic raw cacao nibs
2 large frozen banana, chopped (peel before freezing)
2 cups almond milk
1 tbsp raw organic vanilla bean powder
¼ cup unsweetened shredded coconut, toasted

Cooking Directions
1. Add coffee, milk, cacao nibs, vanilla bean powder, and banana to a blender. Blend until the mixture becomes smooth.
2. Pour even amount of the smoothie into two separate glasses, and top with 2 tablespoons of coconut mixture.

Nutritional Information (Serving Size: 1 cup): Calories: 308, Total Fat: 16g, Saturated Fat: 10g, Cholesterol: 0mg, Sodium: 157mg, Carbohydrates: 46g,

Sweetest Breakfast

This s is a perfect pre-heating smoothie. Make dessert a lot easier to swallow with this delicious guilt-free smoothie! This smoothie is high in fiber and high in tastiness.

Yield: Four Servings
Active Time: 5 minutes
Cooking Time: 0 minutes
Total Time: 5 minutes

Ingredients
1 cup avocado, peeled, seeded, and sliced
1 cup strawberries, sliced
4 pieces organic dark chocolate (85% cacao bar)
1 cup coconut water
2 ½ tbsp organic raw cacao powder
2 tbsp organic raw honey
Ice (if desired)

Cooking Directions
1. Puree coconut water, cacao powder, honey, and dark chocolate in a blender. Blend until all ingredients al pureed and smooth.
2. Add remaining ingredients, and blend until mixture is smooth.

*Note: If mixture becomes too thick, you may need to thin it out by adding water.

Nutritional Information (Serving Size: ¼ of recipe): Calories: 533, Calories from Fat: 267, Total Fat: 30.4g, Saturated Fat: 8.1g, Cholesterol: 0mg, Sodium: 42mg, Carbohydrates: 66.7g, Dietary Fiber: 18.6g, Protein: 8.5g

Smooth and Fruity Italian Ice

This thick homemade ice is a great way to top off your dinner, and a great escape route from any temptation for a high calorie dessert.

Yield: Four Servings
Active Time: 5 minutes
Cooking Time: 0 minutes
Total Time: 5 minutes

Ingredients
2 large frozen banana, chopped (peel before freezing)
2 tbsp coconut, shredded
4 cherries, pitted
1 lime, juiced
1 lemon, juiced
3 cups Ice

Directions
1. Add ice, banana, lemon juice, and lime juice in a blender. Blend at low speed. Continue blending until a smooth consistency is reached.
2. Divide four 8 ounce servings in a tall glass, and garnish each serving with coconut and cherry.
3. Enjoy chilled.

Nutritional Information (Serving Size: 1 cup): Calories: 78, Calories from Fat: 9, Saturated fat: 1g, Cholesterol: 0mg, Sodium: 11mg, Carbohydrates: 21g, Fiber: 4g, Protein: 1g

Strawberry-Banana Soy Smoothie

Try this classic smoothie during anytime of the day!

Yield: One Serving
Active Time: 5 minutes
Cooking Time: 0 minutes
Total Time: 5 minutes

Ingredients
2 cups fresh strawberries, stemmed and halved
1 large frozen banana, chopped (peel before freezing)
1 cups organic soy milk
1 2 tbsp organic raw honey
1 ½ tsp vanilla bean powder

Directions
1. Add all of the ingredients to the blender, and puree until all of the ingredients become completely smooth.
2. Pour into your favorite glass and enjoy!

Nutritional Information (Serving Size: 1 cup): Calories: 78, Calories from Fat: 9, Saturated fat: 1g, Cholesterol: 0mg, Sodium: 24mg, Carbohydrates: 16g, Dietary Fiber: 1g, Protein: 1g

Peanut Butter Blast

Blast away your morning hunger with this protein packed peanut butter shake. This shake is high in fibers, protein, complex cars, antioxidants, and potassium. The incredible taste of this shake might make you forget that you are eating healthy.

Yield: Two Servings
Active Time: 5 minutes
Cooking Time: 0 minutes
Total Time: 5 minutes

Ingredients

2 tbsp organic raw soy protein powder
4 tbsp organic peanut butter
2 tbsp organic raw cacao nibs
2 tbsp cacao powder
½ large frozen banana, chopped (peel before freezing)
1 cup organic almond milk
¼ cup organic rolled oats, cooked
2 ice cubes
Pinch Himalayan Pink Salt

Directions

1. Pour skim milk into the blender, and blend at low speed.
2. Keeping the blender at low speed, add the soy protein powder. Blend for about 30 seconds.
3. Discontinue blending. Add banana, oats, peanut butter, and ice.
4. Mix thoroughly until you reach a smooth, uniform consistency.
5. Pour into your favorite 8 oz. smoothie glass, and enjoy!

Nutritional Information (Serving Size: 1 cup): Calories: 250, Total Fat: 5g, Cholesterol: 222mg, Sodium: 24mg, Carbohydrates: 19g, Dietary Fiber: 4g, Protein: 24g

Creamy Piña Colada

Would you like to have your favorite drink for breakfast without having the hunger and calories afterwards? Then you should definitely try this recipe!

Yield: One Serving
Active Time: 5 minutes
Cooking Time: 0 minutes
Total Time: 5 minutes

Ingredients
2 tsp sweetened coconut, shredded
½ organic rolled oats, cooked
1 cup organic almond milk
⅓ cup fresh pineapple juice
2 tsp vanilla bean powder
1 tbsp organic raw honey
1 tsp monk fruit sweetener

Directions
1. Add all of the ingredients to the blender, and puree until all of the ingredients become completely smooth.
2. Pour into your favorite glass and enjoy!

Nutritional Information (entire recipe): Calories: 271, Total Fat: 8g, Sodium: 347mg, Carbohydrates: 45g, Dietary Fiber: 15g, Protein: 6g

Multi-Melon Protein Smoothie

The various melons give this smoothie a refreshing taste. The CHIA seeds curbs the appetite.

Yield: One Serving
Active Time: 5 minutes
Cooking Time: 0 minutes
Total Time: 5 minutes

Ingredients
2 tbsp organic raw soy protein powder
1 cup organic almond milk
½ cup honeydew, chopped
1 cup watermelon, chopped
1 tbsp chia seeds
1 ½ cup coconut water
Ice (optional)

Directions
1. Pour almond milk into the blender, and blend at low speed.
2. Keeping the blender at low speed, add soy protein powder. Blend for about 30 seconds.
3. Discontinue blending. Add chia seeds, honeydew, watermelon, and ice.
4. Mix thoroughly until you reach a smooth, uniform consistency.
5. Pour into your favorite 16 oz. smoothie glass, and enjoy!

Nutritional Information (entire recipe): Calories: 271, Total Fat: 12g, Sodium: 347mg, Carbohydrates: 45g, Dietary Fiber: 15g, Protein: 26g

Banana Pancakes and Berries

No flour? No problem! This tasty pancake recipe has no need for flour, and will easily replace any crepe recipe in your arsenal. The added berries make the perfect companion to your new favorite breakfast entrée. Rich in pectin, bananas support digestion and gently rids the body of toxins and heavy metals. The delicious fruits also have the ability to increase your alertness, and promotes a healthy brain function.

Yield: Four servings
Active Time: 10 minutes
Cooking Time: 5 minutes
Total Time: 15 minutes

Ingredients
2 large bananas, peeled and chopped
4 eggs
1 tbsp quick oats
½ cup fresh strawberries, sliced
½ cup fresh blueberries
¼ tsp cinnamon
Cooking spray

Directions
1. Place bananas in a large bowl and mash with a potato masher or fork. Beat in eggs, cinnamon, and oats until well combined.
2. Coat a nonstick pan with cooking spray, and place over medium-high heat. Slowly add banana ¼ cup batter to hot pan. Allow each pancake to cook for a minimum of 2 to 3 minutes or until each side is well done.
3. Place each serving onto serving plates and top with ⅛ cup strawberries and ⅛ cup blueberries. Serve immediately.

Nutritional Information (Serving Size: ¼ of recipe): Calories: 125, Total Fat: 5g, Saturated Fat: 1g, Cholesterol: 164mg, Sodium: 10mg, Carbohydrates: 16g, Dietary Fiber: 2g, Protein: 6g

Garbanzo Pancakes

These pancakes are sure to make your breakfast quite intriguing and special. Ditch the refined and bleach flour for the day. Garbanzo flour is the better choice if you want to have a healthy and protein-rich breakfast. Enjoy these pancakes with your favorite breakfast meat to round off the meal. Eating chickpeas frequently can accelerate weight loss, boost intestinal health, and as with most beans, reduce your risk of obtaining type 2 diabetes.

Yield: Four Servings
Active Time: 5 minutes
Cooking Time: 15 minutes
Total Time: 20 minutes

Ingredients
½ cup garbanzo bean flour
¾ cup rolled oats
¼ cup flaxseed meal
½ tsp ground cinnamon
1 cup water
1 tbsp unrefined virgin olive oil

Cooking Directions
1. In a large bowl, mix together flour, oats, flaxseed meal, and cinnamon until the ingredients are fully combined. Slowly add water and stir until mixture becomes smooth.
2. Heat olive oil in a large skillet or on a griddle over medium-high heat. Drop about a spoonful of pancake batter onto the skillet or griddle and allow to cook until the edges of the pancake begin to dry and becomes lightly browned. Turn over pancake and cook on additional side.
3. Repeat for the remaining batter and serve immediately.

Nutritional Information (Serving Size: ¼ of recipe): Calories: 133, Calories from Fat: 17, Total Fat: 1.9g, Saturated Fat: 0.2g, Cholesterol: 0mg, Sodium: 125mg, Carbohydrates: 24.5g, Dietary Fiber: 2.5g, Protein: 4.9g

Sweet and Creamy Vanilla Multi-grain Hot Cereal

Try this hot and healthy cereal and kick-out those refined, HIGH SUGAR cereals. Meant to be made the night before, this slow cooker recipe will surely become one of your favorite breakfast meals. Last for up to five days when refrigerated, or up to three months when frozen.

Yield: Four Servings
Active Time: 5 minutes
Cooking Time: 7 hours
Total Time: 7 hours, 5 minutes

Ingredients
¾ cup steel-cut oats
¾ cup pearl barley
½ cup quinoa, rinsed
6 cups organic unsweetened plain almond milk
2 cups organic coconut water
¼ cup raw organic honey
½ tsp Himalayan Pink Salt

Cooking Directions
1. In a slow-cooker that measures up to about a gallon or a gallon and a half, mix together milk, coconut water, honey, and salt.
2. Gently stir in oats, barley, and quinoa. Place lid over the slow-cooker and ingredients on low heat for a minimum of 5 to 7 hours or until all grains are tender.
3. Serve immediately.

Nutritional Information (Serving Size: ¾ cup): Calories: 160, Calories from Fat: 25, Total Fat: 3g, Saturated Fat: 0g, Cholesterol: 0mg, Sodium: 230mg, Carbohydrates: 30g, Dietary Fiber: 4g, Protein: 5g

Crispy Eggplant Bacon

America's obsession with bacon is obvious, but the consumption of pork has no healthy outcome in the long-run. On average, Americans consume about 5,760,000,000 pounds of bacon each year. However, there is an alternative to this bacon craze that is plaguing the country, EGGLANT strips. This recipe will make bacon a no-contender, and will hopefully make you forget about bacon for good! You can store leftovers for up to three days at room temperature.

Yield: Eight Servings
Active Time: 10 minutes
Cooking Time: 1 hour, 30 minutes
Total Time: 3 hour, 40 minutes

Ingredients
1 large eggplant (16 ounces), quartered vertically and thinly sliced
1 ½ tsp Himalayan Pink Salt
¼ cup pure cane sugar
2 tbsp organic apple cider vinegar
1 tbsp unrefined virgin olive oil
½ tsp smoked paprika
⅛ tsp ground chipotle

Cooking Directions
1. Add eggplant to a large colander and season with salt. Allow the eggplants to drain for about 1 hour. Rinse and pat the eggplant dry.
2. Mix together ¼ cup water, vinegar, olive oil, sugar, paprika, and chipotle in a shallow baking dish. Place eggplant into the baking dish and allow the eggplant to marinate for another hour. Stir occasionally.
3. Set oven to 250 degrees, and lightly grease 2 baking sheets with olive oil.
4. Place each marinated eggplant strip onto the baking sheets in one even layer. Bake the eggplant for a minimum of 1 hour and 30 minute or until the eggplant strips have become dry and golden brown.
5. Remove from oven and allow the eggplant to cool before serving.

Nutritional Information (Serving Size: 6 slices): Calories: 40, Calories from Fat: 10, Total Fat: 1g, Saturated Fat: 0g, Cholesterol: 0mg, Sodium: 80mg, Carbohydrates: 8g, Dietary Fiber: 2g, Protein: 1g

Paleo Avocado in a Basket

Avocado has a high concentration of monounsaturated fats. Monounsaturated fats are considered among one of the healthiest fats. Diets that are high in monounsaturated fats and contain a low amount of low-quality carbs has been proven to help improve insulin sensitivity. This is quick and easy high protein breakfast that is a pretty cool, gluten-free variation of the traditional egg in a basket recipe, and is one of the best ways to start your day off right.

Yield: One servings
Active Time: 5 minutes
Cooking Time: 10 minutes
Total Time: 15 minutes

Ingredients
1 avocado, halved, pitted, and peeled
2 free range organic eggs
1 tsp Unrefined Virgin Coconut Oil
2 tsp fresh parsley
1 tsp Himalayan Pink Salt
1 tsp fresh ground black pepper

Cooking Directions
1. Heat and melt coconut oil in a medium skillet, and place the avocado in the skillet (pitted side down).
2. Crack the egg and pour into the pit of the avocado. Season with salt and pepper and allow to cook for about 2 to 5 minutes or until the bottom of the avocado begins to become firm.
3. Flip over the avocado and cook for an additional 3 minutes or until the egg is set to your desire.
4. Repeat with the remaining avocado half.
5. Place both avocado halves on a serving plate and garnish with parsley. Serve immediately.

Nutritional Information: Calories: 645, Calories from Fat: 54g, Saturated Fat: 22g, Cholesterol: 372mg, Sodium: 2,231mg, Potassium: 1,253mg, Carbohydrate: 26g, Protein: 19.7g

Seed Crunch Bunch

This simple walnut and seed mix is a great way to start you're day and perfect for those busy mornings.

Yield: Sixteen servings
Active Time: 10 minutes
Cooking Time: 10 minutes
Total Time: 50 minutes

Ingredients
1 cup pumpkin seeds, hulled
1 cup sunflower seeds
2 tbsp sesame seeds
¾ cup dried cranberries
1 ½ cup walnuts
½ cup brown sugar

Directions
1. In a medium saucepan, melt brown sugar over medium-low heat. Add walnuts and sesame seeds and stir until walnuts are coated with the sugar and seeds. Set to the side.
2. Mix together coated walnuts, pumpkin seeds, sunflower seeds, and cranberries in a bowl.
3. Serve immediately or enjoy later.

Nutritional Information: Calories: 230, Calories from Fat: 10, Saturated fat: 1g, Cholesterol: 0mg, Sodium: 257mg, Carbohydrates: 7.3g, Fiber: 10g, Protein: 7g

Sweet Nutty Snack Mix

Cousin to the peach and apricot, the almond is a seed (not a nut) that carries many health benefits that pack a powerful punch. Almonds contain bad-ass phytochemicals that help avert certain types of cancer. Increasing your consumption of nuts will also reduce the risk of developing gallstones, and decreases cholesterol.

Yield: Seventeen servings
Active Time: 25 minutes
Cooking Time: 20 minutes
Total Time: 45 minutes

Ingredients
1 cup slivered almonds
1 cup unsalted cashews
1 cup unsalted pumpkinseed kernels
1 large egg white
¼ monk fruit sweetener
1 tsp ground chipotle chili pepper
½ tsp ground cumin
½ tsp dried oregano
½ tsp chili powder
Salt to taste

Directions
1. Preheat oven to 325 degrees.
2. Combine sweetener, salt, chipotle, cumin, oregano, and chili powder in a small bowl. Mix well to combine and set spice mixture aside.
3. Beat egg white in a separate bowl until foamy and add almonds, cashews, and pumpkin seeds. Gently toss to coat and sprinkle with spice mixture.
4. Line a baking sheet with parchment paper and spread nut mixture evenly out onto baking sheet.
5. Bake mixture for 15 minutes or until nuts are lightly toasted and browned. Stirring once, immediately return pan to oven for an additional 15 minutes, but turn oven off.
6. Allow to cool before serving.

Nutritional Information (Serving Size: 3 tbsp snack mix): Calories: 130, Calories from Fat: 9.7, Saturated fat: 1.4g, Cholesterol: 0mg, Sodium: 175mg, Carbohydrates: 7.3g, Fiber: 1.1g, Protein: 4.5g

Quick Fruit Mix

You can't go wrong with fruit and yogurt.

Yield: Four servings
Active Time: 15 minutes
Cooking Time: 0 minutes
Total Time: 45 minutes

Ingredients
1 nectarine, pitted and chopped
1 large orange, peeled and cut into chunks
1 apple, cored and chopped
½ cup grapes
¼ cup fresh orange juice
6 tbsp plain low-fat yogurt

Directions
1. Combine apple, orange, nectarine, and grape in a large bowl. Pour orange juice over the fruit mixture. Toss well and allow mixture to chill in fridge for 30 minutes.
2. When ready to serve, evenly divide servings, place in desired serving dish or glass, and top with a dollop of yogurt.

Nutritional Information (Serving Size: ¼ of recipe): Calories: 90, Calories from Fat: 7, Saturated fat: 0.3g, Cholesterol: 1mg, Sodium: 17mg, Carbohydrates: 20.6g, Fiber: 2.7g, Protein: 2.3g

Skillet Asparagus Salad with Goat Cheese

Asparagus is a brain healthy food that aids our brain against cognitive decline. Similar to the abilities of leafy greens, asparagus contains high amounts of folate which works with vitamin B12. Making the decision to eat asparagus is a great idea, and this recipe makes the idea an even better one.

Yield: Four servings
Active Time: 15 minutes
Cooking Time: 0 minutes
Total Time: 45 minutes

Ingredients
1 ½ pound asparagus spears, trimmed (about 30 spears)
2 cups mixed baby salad greens
½ cup goat cheese, crumbled
3 tbsp toasted pecans, chopped
1 tsp monk fruit sweetener
1 tbsp dry white wine
1 ½ fresh lemon juice
1 cup water
½ Dijon mustard
2 tsp orange rind, thinly cut
1 tsp lemon rind, thinly cut
¼ cup fresh orange juice
1 tbsp fresh tarragon leaves, finely chopped
1 tsp fresh parsley, finely chopped
6 tsp unrefined virgin olive oil (divided)
Salt and pepper to taste

Directions
1. In a large bowl combine, salt and pepper to taste, asparagus, and olive oil and toss gently to coat asparagus.
2. Over medium-high heat, sauté asparagus mixture for 4 minutes or until each spear is lightly charred and crisp. Stir occasionally. Remove from heat and set aside.
3. Microwave 1 cup of water on HIGH in microwave for 2 minutes or just until water begins to bubble. Remove from microwave and add orange and lemon rind. Allow to stand for at least 20 seconds and drain.
4. In a small saucepan, stir orange juice, rind mixture, and sweetener and bring to a boil over medium heat. Immediately reduce heat to low, and cook for 5 minutes until the mixture reduces to at 3 tbsp. Set aside.
5. In a medium bowl, mix together wine, lemon juice, remaining olive oil, orange juice mixture, mustard, and salt and pepper to taste. Stirring slowly with a whisk.
6. Serve immediately.

Nutritional Information (Serving Size: ⅓ cup greens, 5 asparagus spears, 1 ½ tsp pecan, and 4 tsp cheese): Calories: 117, Calories from Fat: 8.4g, Saturated Fat: 2.2g, Cholesterol: 4mg, Sodium: 152mg, Carbohydrates: 7g, Fiber: 3g, Protein: 5g

Refreshing Watermelon Salad

This tasty and fresh salad will make any lunch special. This salad features cubed watermelon, red onion, Kalamata olives, mint, and feta cheese.

Yield: Four servings
Active Time: 10 minutes
Cooking Time: 0 minutes
Total Time: 70 minutes

Ingredients
½ cantaloupe, peeled and seeded
1 ½ large cucumbers
½ honeydew melon
1 ½ pounds watermelon, seeded and cubed
¼ cup Kalamata olives, pitted
½ cup red onion, chopped
½ cup feta cheese, crumbled
3 tbsp lime juice
¼ cup fresh parsley, finely chopped
¼ cup fresh mint, finely chopped

Directions
1. In a medium bowl, combine lime juice and onion, and allow to stand for 10 minutes. Mix in watermelon, olives, parsley, and mint. Cover with plastic wrap and allow to chill for 1 hour.

Nutritional Information (Serving Size: ½ cup of salad and about 1 ½ tsp cheese): Calories: 46, Calories from Fat: 23g, Saturated fat: 0.9g, Cholesterol: 4mg, Sodium: 136mg, Carbohydrates: 5.5g, Fiber: 0.5g, Protein: 1.2g

Quinoa Chard Pilaf

Quinoa is definitely a better alternative to that plain old rice. Enjoying quinoa as a pilaf will deplete rice's significance from your diet. Quinoa is a gluten-free, organically grown crop which means is GMO FREE! High in fiber and complete proteins, you can always bet on quinoa to provide you with the best nutrients, and to be the compliment to your favorite meal.

Yield: Four Servings
Active Time: 20 minutes
Cooking Time: 20 minutes
Total Time: 40 minutes

Ingredients
1 ½ tsp olive oil
½ onion, diced
1 ½ cloves garlic, minced
1 cup uncooked quinoa, rinsed
½ cup canned lentils, rinsed
4 ounces fresh mushrooms, chopped
2 cups vegetable broth
½ bunch Swiss chard, stems removed and shredded

Directions
1. In a large pot, heat olive oil over medium-high heat. Add garlic and onions and sauté until onions are tender, or for at least 5 minutes.
2. Stir in quinoa, lentils, mushrooms and vegetable broth. Cover and allow to cook for 20 minutes.
3. Remove pot from stove. Add chard into pot and stir.
4. Cover pot and allow to cook until chard has wilted, or for 5 minutes.

Nutritional Information (Serving Size ¼ of recipe): Calories: 224, Calories from Fat: 42, Saturated fat: 0.6g, Cholesterol: 0mg, Sodium: 323mg, Carbohydrates: 36.6g, Fiber: 6.2g, Protein: 9.6g

Cabbage and Apple Salad

Cabbage and apples may not sound too appetizing. Try this dish, and you'll be surprised at how much you love it.

Yield: Two servings
Active Time: 10 minutes
Cooking Time: 10 minutes
Total Time: 20 minutes

Ingredients
4 cups green cabbage, sliced
1 cups apple, sliced
½ tsp caraway seeds
1 ½ tbsp unrefined virgin olive oil

Directions
1. In a large pan, heat olive oil and canola oil over medium-high heat.
2. Combine cabbage, apple, and caraway seed in skillet and allow to cook for 5 minutes covered.
3. Uncover and cook until cabbage and apples are tender or for at least 5 minutes, stirring occasionally.

Nutritional Information (Serving Size: 1 cup): Calories: 73, Total Fat: 3.7g, Saturated: 1.4g, Monounsaturated: 1.5g, Polyunsaturated Fat: 0.6g, Protein: 1.4g, Carbohydrate: 10.3g, Fiber: 2.9g, Cholesterol: 5mg, Iron: 0.5mg, Sodium: 214mg, Calcium: 42mg

High Protein Egg and Salmon Sandwich

Egg whites and salmon on a toasted whole-wheat English muffin is the perfect way to begin your morning! This flavorful protein rich sandwich, packed with Omega-3s is a great way to BREAK the FAST, and satisfy your hunger. Add a piece of fruit or a glass of all natural juice, to make this meal more filling.

Yield: Four servings
Active Time: 14 minutes
Cooking Time: 3 minutes
Total Time: 17 minutes

Ingredients
4 ounces wild-caught smoked salmon
4 large organic eggs
4 (1 ounce) slices organic rye bread, toasted
¼ cup low-fat cream cheese
2 tbsp red onion, minced
1 tbsp dill, chopped
1 cup fresh arugula
4 cups water
Parsley and pepper to taste

Directions
1. In a large cast-iron skillet, bring water and vinegar to a simmer over medium heat. Carefully add eggs one at a time. Allow eggs to simmer to desired doneness or for a minimum of 3 minutes. Remove from heat and set aside.
2. Assemble sandwiches by layering cheese, onion, and parsley and pepper over a single slice of bread. Top with ¼ cup arugula and 1 ounce of salmon.
3. Using a slotted spoon, carefully remove poached eggs from skillet and top each sandwiched with egg.

Nutritional Information (Serving Size 1 sandwich): Calories: 219, Total Fat: 11g, Saturated Fat: 4.1g, Cholesterol: 228mg, Sodium: 649mg, Carbohydrates: 14.4g, Dietary Fiber: 2.3g, Protein: 16.5g

Grilled Salmon with Spaghetti Squash and Pecan Salad

Salmon is one of those "flexible" fish that allows you to pair it with anything you want, and still come out with a good dish. This recipe combines salmon and a warm spaghetti squash and pecan salad that gives this dish an incredible flavor, crunch, and nuttiness.

Yield: Four Servings
Active Time: 30 minutes
Cooking Time: 55 minutes
Total Time: 85 minutes

Ingredients
4 wild-caught salmon fillets (Each fillet should be about 6 ounces)
3 cups spaghetti squash, diced
1 cup celery leaves
1 cup yellow onion, thinly sliced
3 cloves garlic, divided (2 crushed separately and 1 sliced)
¼ cup pecan halves, toasted
¼ cup toasted almond halves, toasted
1 ½ tbsp fresh lemon juice
½ cup fresh parsley, coarsely chopped
1 tbsp garlic cloves, minced
2 sprigs fresh thyme
1 cup unrefined virgin olive oil (divided)
Himalayan Pink Salt and freshly ground black pepper to taste
Cooking spray

Directions
1. Set oven to 375 degrees and coat a large baking sheet with cooking spray and set to the side.
2. Toss together squash, 1 crushed garlic clove, 1 tablespoon of olive oil, and thyme in a large bowl. Be sure all ingredients are well coated with the olive oil.
3. Dump and spread out the squash mixture onto the prepared baking sheet. Season with salt and pepper and bake in preheated oven for a minimum of 40 minutes. The squash should be tender. Remove from oven and allow the squash to rest. (****It is recommended to occasionally stir squash to avoid scorching.*)
4. Add 2 tablespoons olive oil, celery leaves, parsley, lemon juice, salt, pepper, and remaining clove of crushed garlic to a blender or food processor. Blend until all the ingredients are well combined and finely chopped. Set pesto sauce to the side.
5. Prepare your grill to your preferred temperature.
6. Coat salmon fillets with a layer of olive oil, salt, and pepper. Slowly add seasoned salmon fillets to the prepared grill (skin side

down) and grill for a minimum of 5 seconds or until the fish is easily flaked with a fork. Turn off the grill and allow the fish to rest, but keep warm.
7. Sauté sliced garlic and onion in a large pan over high heat. Season with salt and pepper and simmer until the onions begin to caramelize. Mix in squash, almonds, and pecans. Simmer for an additional 3 minutes. Remove from heat.
8. Serve each salmon fillet with a side of the squash and pecan salad topped with the pesto dressing.

Nutritional Facts: Calories: 508, Total Fat: 31.8g, Saturated Fat: 5.3g, Protein: 38.6g, Carbohydrate: 18.8g, Dietary Fiber: 4.2g, Cholesterol: 100mg, Sodium: 431mg

Tasty Tomato and Beet Salad

Heirloom tomatoes are some of the most beautiful fruits out there, and probably has graced you with its presence a thousand times. However, what most people don't know about heirloom tomatoes is that they come in an assortment of colors, and not just your ordinary red. We encourage you to expand your "tomato palette" by using heirloom tomatoes that vary in color. Not only will this make your salad VERY colorful, but it will also be more appeasing to the eye! Since tomatoes are high in Vitamin C, you can count on your immune system to gain some added strength.

Yield: Six Servings
Active Time: 15 minutes
Cooking Time: 1 hour, 15 minutes
Total Time: 1 hour, 30 minutes

Ingredients
2 medium organic red beets, roots trimmed and stems removed
2 medium organic golden beets, roots trimmed and stems removed
2 pounds heirloom tomatoes, sliced (red or varying colors)
3 cups heirloom cherry tomatoes, halved
1 ½ cup organic feta cheese, crumbled
2 tbsp red wine vinegar
2 tsp basil pesto sauce
1 tbsp capers
3 tbsp fresh chives, chopped
2 tbsp fresh tarragon, chopped
1 tbsp shallots, chopped
2 tbsp cloves of garlic, minced
3 tbsp unrefined virgin olive oil
Himalayan Pink Salt and freshly ground black pepper

Directions
1. Set the oven to 400 degrees.
2. Poke each of the beets with a fork, and wrap in foil. Bake for about one hour or until the beets become soft. Remove beets from oven and allow to cool. Slice the cooked beets into about 18 slices that are at least ¼" thick.
3. In a small bowl, combine chives, tarragon, shallots, garlic, capers, olive oil, vinegar, and pesto.
4. In a separate bowl, add tomatoes and 5 tsp of mustard mixture. Toss lightly to coat.
5. Arrange 3 beet slices, ½ cup cherry tomatoes, and 4 tomato slices evenly between each serving. Drizzle each plate with about 3 teaspoon of leftover mustard mixture. Garnish each plate with cherry tomatoes and ¼ cup feta cheese. Sprinkle with salt and pepper to taste.

Nutritional Facts (Serving Size: 3 beet slices, 4 tomato slices, ½ cup cherry tomatoes, and ¼ cup feta cheese): Calories: 207, Total

Fat: 14g, Saturated Fat: 5.5g, Cholesterol: 15mg, Sodium: 625mg, Carbohydrates: 40g, Dietary Fiber: 4g, Protein: 8g

Sweet Black Bean Burrito

Here is a delectable vegetarian burrito with a noticeably sweet taste. Sweet potatoes are loaded with vitamin A, fiber, and potassium. Pairing the sweet potatoes with the black beans makes this burrito one of the healthiest burritos around.

Yield: Eight Servings
Active Time: 30 minutes
Cooking Time: 45 minutes
Total Time: 1 hour, 15 minutes

Ingredients
5 cups peeled cubed sweet potatoes
12 whole-grain flour tortillas (about 10" in diameter)
3 ½ cups onions, diced
4 garlic cloves, minced
1 tbsp fresh green chili pepper, minced
4 tsp ground cumin
4 tsp ground coriander
4 ½ cups cooked black beans
⅔ cup cilantro leaf, finely chopped
2 tbsp fresh lemon juice
2 tsp unrefined virgin olive oil
1 ½ tsp Himalayan Pink Salt
Fresh salsa

Cooking Directions
1. Set oven to 350 degrees, and lightly grease a baking dish. Set to the side.
2. Boil sweet potatoes in salted water in a medium saucepan for about 10 minutes or until the potatoes are tender. Remove from heat, drain, and set to the side.
3. Heat olive oil in a medium skillet over medium-low heat. Toss in onions, chili, and garlic. Saute until the onions become tender and transparent or for about 7 minutes. Stir in cumin and coriander and simmer for an additional 2 to 3 minutes. Stir often. Discontinue cooking and set to the side.
4. Add black beans, cilantro, lemon juice, salt, and sweet potatoes to a food processor. Blend until the ingredients are pulverized and smooth. Pour into a large bowl and stir in onion mixture.
5. Add about ⅔ to ¾ cup of the sweet potato mixture to each tortilla. Gently roll up the tortilla and place into the baking dish seam side down.
6. Once all tortilla have been assembled and added to the baking dish, cover the dish with foil and bake for about 30 minutes. Serve hot and top with desired amount of salsa.

Variations
- Substitute tortillas with wonton skins to lighten up the dish.
- Garnish with a nice amount of guacamole for nice touch of creaminess.

Nutritional Information: Calories: 575, Calories from Fat: 92, Total Fat: 10.3g, Saturated: 2.2g, Protein: 19.8g, Carbohydrate: 101.9g, Dietary Fiber: 15.9g, Cholesterol: 0.0mg, Sodium: 1156.3mg

Vegetarian Stuffed Red Bell Peppers

Stuffed bell peppers is such a versatile dish. You can pretty much stuff a bell pepper with anything you like. Our choice of stuffing for this recipe is vegetables, legumes, and rice. However, you are welcome to add your own ingredients. Just make sure the ingredients you add are healthy to make your recipe a winner!

Yield: Four servings
Active Time: 20 minutes
Cooking Time: 60 minutes
Total Time: 80 minutes

Ingredients
4 red bell peppers, tops and seeds removed
1 cup brown rice, uncooked
2 cups black-eyed peas, cooked, rinsed, and drained
2 ¼ cup water
¼ onions, chopped
4 tbsp fresh chives, finely chopped
2 cloves, chopped
2 cup spinach, chopped
1 tsp unrefined virgin olive oil
Himalayan Pink Salt and ground black pepper to taste

Directions
1. Set oven to 350 degrees.
2. Over high heat, bring water and brow rice to a boil in a medium sauce pan. Decrease heat to medium-low, and cover. Allow rice to simmer for 45 to 50 minutes or until tender. Remove rice from heat and set to the side.
3. Coat a baking sheet with cooking spray, and arrange bell peppers on sheet. Bake bell peppers for about 15 minutes, or until tender. Remove bell peppers from oven, and set the bell peppers to the side to allow the flesh to rest.
4. Add olive oil, onion, and garlic to a large pan. Sauté vegetables over medium heat for about 5 minutes or until onion becomes slightly transparent. Mix in black-eyed peas and spinach. Simmer for a minimum of 5 to 8 minutes or until the spinach has wilted. Add the cooked brown rice. Season with salt and pepper to taste.
5. Gently stuff the rice and veggie mixture into each bell. Garnish each bell pepper with 1 tbsp of chives and serve immediately.

Nutritional Facts (Serving Size: 1 stuffed bell pepper): Calories: 271, Calories from Fat: 29, Saturated fat: 0.6g, Cholesterol: 0mg, Sodium: 472mg, Carbohydrates: 51.4g, Fiber: 8.5g, Protein: 9.5g

Grilled Fiesta Fish Tacos with Lime-Yogurt Sauce

Fish tacos are already delicious, but add the smokiness of the grill and you will have one phenomenal fish taco.

Yield: Six Servings
Active Time: 15 minutes
Cooking Time: 20 minutes
Total Time: 35 minutes

Ingredients
2 pounds wild-caught tilapia, sliced into 1" strips
12 organic whole-grain tortillas
1 ½ cup red cabbage, shredded
2 large tomatoes, chopped
½ cup salsa
2 limes, quartered
3 tbsp lime juice, freshly squeezed (3 limes)
1 cup plain Greek yogurt
1 tsp ground cumin
1 garlic clove, minced
1 bunch fresh cilantro, chopped
Unrefined virgin olive oil
Himalayan Pink Salt and ground black pepper to taste

Cooking Directions
1. Lightly grease grill with olive oil and set to medium heat or at about 450 degrees.
2. Sprinkle tilapia with salt and pepper; place onto the heated grill. Cook fish for a minimum of 2 to 3 minutes per side until thoroughly cooked.
3. In the meantime, warm tortillas up on the grill, turning constantly. Remove tortillas from heat and set to the side. Keep warm.
4. In a medium bowl, combine lime juice, yogurt, cumin, garlic, cilantro, salt, and pepper. Stir until all ingredients are well combined and set to the side.
5. Once fish is done grilling, arrange about 3 fish strips onto a tortilla, top with tomatoes, red cabbage, and a spoonful of yogurt sauce. Garnish each serving with a lime wedge and about a tbsp of salsa. Serve immediately.

Nutritional Information (Serving Size: 2 tacos): Calories: 617.6, Total Fat: 12g, Saturated Fat: 5g, Cholesterol: 110mg, Sodium: 1294.8mg, Carbohydrates: 66.2g, Dietary Fiber: 8g, Protein: 61.8g

Mesquite Collard Greens

This smoky and meatless collard greens recipe is bound to have you coming back for seconds, and that's ok due to its low-calorie content. You can never lose with leafy greens anyway.

Yield: Six Servings
Active Time: 5 minutes
Cooking Time: 50 minutes
Total Time: 55 minutes

Ingredients
1 large yellow onion, halved and thinly sliced
½ tsp red chile flakes
3 garlic cloves, chopped
1 ½ pound collard greens, stems removed, leaves roughly torn, and rinsed
⅓ cup red wine vinegar
1 tbsp smoked paprika
⅛ tsp Himalayan Pink Salt
½ tsp ground black pepper

Cooking Directions
1. In a large pan sauté onions over medium-high heat form a minimum of 2 minutes. Stir frequently. Mix in 2 tbsp water, red pepper flakes, and garlic. Allow onion mixture to cook for 3 minutes or until the onion becomes slightly transparent.
2. Stirring constantly, mix in collard greens and allow to simmer for a minimum of 5 minutes. Toss in vinegar, paprika, salt, pepper and 2 cups of water. Slowly bring greens mixtures to a boil and then immediately reduce the heat.
3. Simmer the greens for a minimum of 40 to 45 minutes or until the greens become tender and the water has evaporated.

Nutritional Information: Calories: 45, Calories from Fat: 5, Total Fat: 0g, Saturated Fat: 0g, Cholesterol: 0mg, Sodium: 85mg, Carbohydrates: 10g, Dietary Fiber: 4g, Protein: 3g

Salmon Cakes with Chervil and Green Bean Salad

Yield: Four Servings
Active Time: 45 minutes
Cooking Time: 40 minutes
Total Time: 1 hour, 35 minutes

Ingredients
Salmon Cakes:
7 ounces wild-caught salmon
2 cups saltine crackers, finely crushed
2 green onions, finely chopped
1 organic egg, lightly beaten
1 tbsp unrefined virgin olive oil
Cooking spray

Salad:
1 ¾ cup green beans, topped, tailed, blanched, cooled, and drained
4 ½ ounces watercress
1 (14 ounce) can artichoke hearts, drained and halved
16 small black olives, pitted and chopped
⅔ cup cherry tomatoes, halved
3 tbsp fresh parsley, finely chopped
2 tsp lemon thyme
1 tbsp fennel fronds, chopped
3 tbsp chervil, chopped
Unrefined virgin olive oil
Himalayan Pink Salt and freshly ground black pepper

Dressing:
5 tbsp unrefined virgin olive oil
½ garlic clove, crushed
1 ½ tbsp balsamic vinegar

Cooking Directions
Salmon Cakes:
1. Preheat oven to 350 degrees, and a large nonstick baking sheet with cooking spray.
2. Arrange the salmon on prepared baking sheet skin side down, brush with olive oil, and season with salt and pepper. Bake in preheated oven until fish is cooked through or for a minimum of 15 to 20 minutes.
3. Remove fish from oven, wrap in foil, and place in fridge to rest and cool. Fish should be removed when cold.
4. Increase the oven temperature to 375 degrees, and prepare a baking sheet with cooking spray. Set to the side.
5. Remove chilled salmon from fridge and flake. Add flaked salmon, egg, olive oil, green onions, ⅔ cup cracker crumbs, and lemon pepper to taste in a medium bowl. Mix ingredients well to

combine and form into eight patties. Cover the patties with the remaining cracker crumbs, and arrange on prepared baking sheet.
6. Bake salmon cakes for a minimum of 10 minutes or until both sides of each patty is browned on each side. Flip patties occasionally to ensure even cooking. Remove from oven and set to the side. Keep warm.

Salad:
1. Add green beans to a large shallow bowl. Sprinkle with 1 ½ tablespoon parsley, lemon thyme, fennel, and a drizzle of olive oil. Toss well to evenly coat green beans. Top beans with watercress, chervil, artichoke hearts, olives, tomatoes, and spring onion.

Dressing:
1. Add olive oil, balsamic vinegar, and garlic into a small bowl. Season with salt and pepper, and whisk well until ingredients become emulsified.
2. Pour dressing over salad and toss to coat the entire salad.
3. Serve salad with two salmon cakes. Enjoy!

Nutritional Information (Serving Size: 2 salmon cakes and 1 ⅔ cup salad): Calories: 388, Total Fat: 14g, Saturated Fat: 2g, Cholesterol: 74mg, Sodium: 797mg, Carbohydrates: 65g, Dietary Fiber: 10g, Protein: 22g

CONCLUSION:

I hope this book has provided you with the information essential to adopting a more healthy diet. I Practice what I preach and I can tell you that I have personally tried every single recipe in this book but two of them. The increased energy you feel after eating a healthy snack, or indulging in an energizing smoothie is truly phenomenal. I love sharing my health knowledge with others and I honestly hope that this book will revolutionize the way you eat, hence revolutionizing the way you feel on a daily basis. Cheers to your health!

Other books by Ariana Hunter:

"Dating, Flirting & Everything in Between: Flirt Fearlessly, Date Deeper and Exude Confidence, While Being Yourself!"

"A Woman's Guide to Living a More Fulfilling Life: Find Your Happiness, Unlock Your Passions, Make All the Right Choices and Love the Woman You Are"

If you would like to be notified whenever I have a new book coming out, or whenever one of my books goes up on free promotion, feel free to drop me a quick line at a_hunter2015@hotmail.com. I do not believe in spam mail and I promise to only use your email address to help you better your life ☺

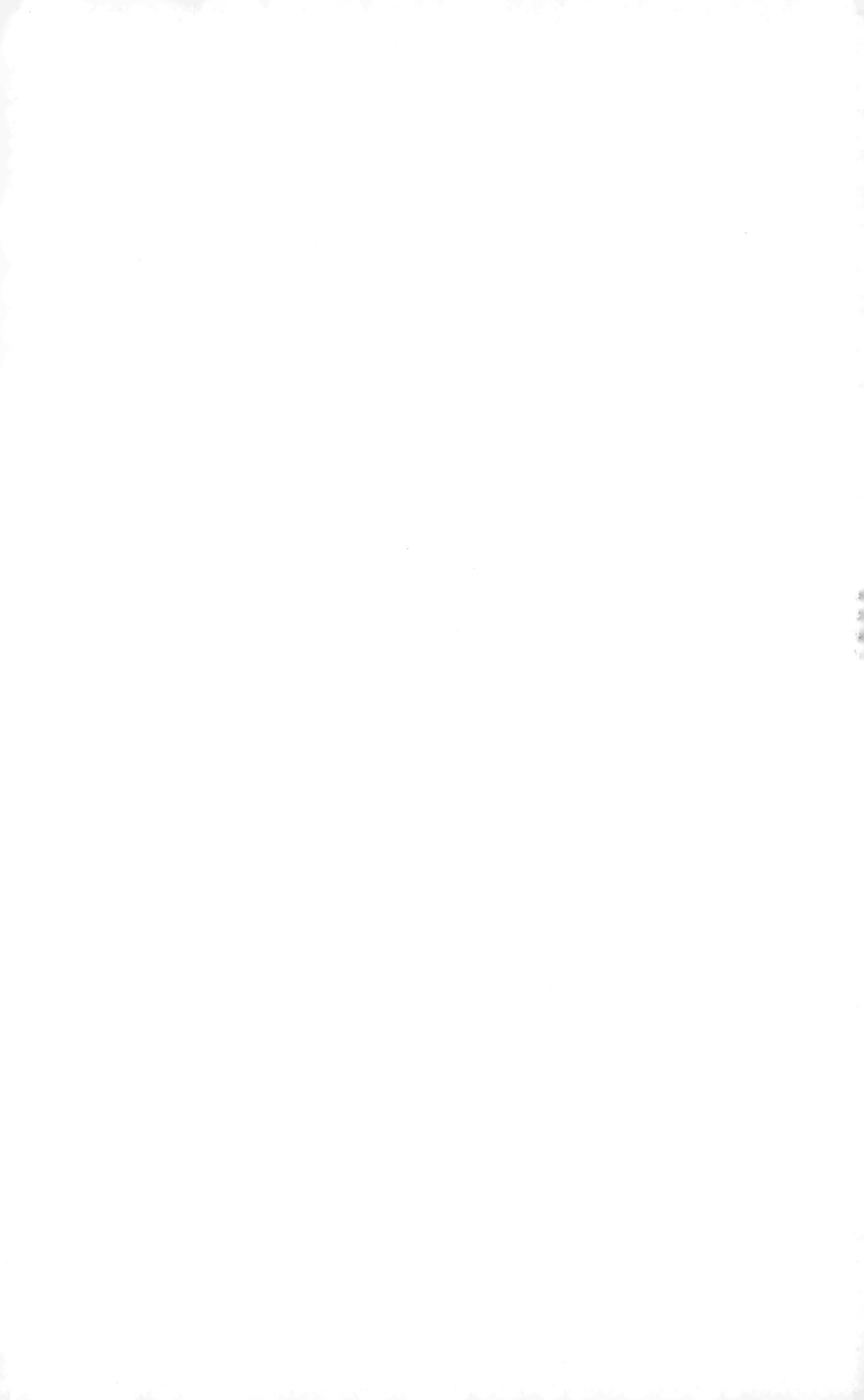

Printed in Great Britain
by Amazon